YOUR KNOWLEDGE HAS VALUE

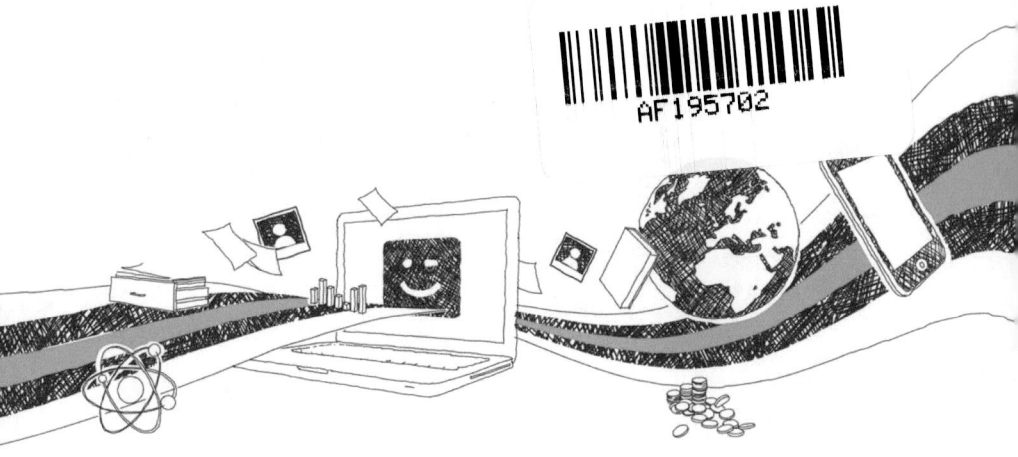

- We will publish your bachelor's and master's thesis, essays and papers

- Your own eBook and book - sold worldwide in all relevant shops

- Earn money with each sale

Upload your text at www.GRIN.com
and publish for free

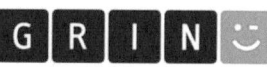

Bibliographic information published by the German National Library:

The German National Library lists this publication in the National Bibliography; detailed bibliographic data are available on the Internet at http://dnb.dnb.de .

This book is copyright material and must not be copied, reproduced, transferred, distributed, leased, licensed or publicly performed or used in any way except as specifically permitted in writing by the publishers, as allowed under the terms and conditions under which it was purchased or as strictly permitted by applicable copyright law. Any unauthorized distribution or use of this text may be a direct infringement of the author s and publisher s rights and those responsible may be liable in law accordingly.

Imprint:

Copyright © 2018 GRIN Verlag
Print and binding: Books on Demand GmbH, Norderstedt Germany
ISBN: 9783668615809

This book at GRIN:

https://www.grin.com/document/387501

Patrick Kimuyu

Ethical issues regarding the charging of overweight people on airplanes. The "pay-by-weight" policy

GRIN Verlag

GRIN - Your knowledge has value

Since its foundation in 1998, GRIN has specialized in publishing academic texts by students, college teachers and other academics as e-book and printed book. The website www.grin.com is an ideal platform for presenting term papers, final papers, scientific essays, dissertations and specialist books.

Visit us on the internet:

http://www.grin.com/

http://www.facebook.com/grincom

http://www.twitter.com/grin_com

Introduction

Debates over ethical issues do not seem to end anytime soon. Over the past half century, ethical issues have been emerging in the global society, especially the industrialized world. For instance, the debate over the decriminalization of abortion and euthanasia has lingered around for quite too long without a consensus decision. On the other hand, the issue of gay marriages that emerge in 1970s remained surrounded by immense controversy until a few months ago when the US Supreme Court brought the issue to rest through upholding gay rights. Surprisingly, the termination of gay marriages debate did not seem to change the course of ethical phenomena among the global society. Recently, a new ethical issue emerged: the pay-as-you-weigh policy. This policy requires obese people to pay extra charge in the airlines. In retrospect, obesity is considered as an ethical issue and it has emerged to be a controversial subject (Funke, 2009). It is an ethical issue because it causes adverse consequences to obese individuals, as well as, the society. However, these factors do not seem to be part of the justification for the introduction of pay-as-you-weigh pricing in the aviation industry. Instead, the core argument by airline administrators and economists is that flying obese people increases fuel costs; thus, the so-called 'fat-taxes' will address the issue of financial costs. Contrary to this perspective held within the aviation industry, environmentalists view obesity as an issue that has environmental cost. The increased fuel consumption by airplanes is believed to exacerbate climate change, primarily global warming due to increased greenhouse gas emissions (Singer, 2012). From these perspectives, it is apparent that obesity is a controversial issue. Therefore, this research will provide a comprehensive overview of the ethical issue of charging overweight people on airlines.

Overview of the 'Pay-by-Weight' on Airlines

Ordinarily, airlines have been charging passengers as per seats rather than their body weight. However, this approach began experiencing opposition in the past decade. It is imperative that the airline industry is entangled in the globalization paradox (Thomas, 2011). The idea of charging passengers based on their weight emerged after economists in the aviation industry discovered a significant increase in fuel cost that was attributable to flying obese people.

In a nutshell, the issue of introducing 'pay-by-weight' system in the aviation industry has been sparked by the arguments of just three experts: Tony Webber, Bharat P. Bhatta and Peter Singer. It is apparent that opinions of these experts have influenced the way in which airlines view pricing of flights.

It all began with Tony Webber, who investigated changes in average body weight of people flying with Qantas, the Australian airline. Webber, who worked with the airline as the chief economist identified average weight increase since 2000 and calculated the correlated fuel cost. In his findings, he noticed that the average weight of adults increased by two kilograms; thus, increasing fuel cost. He interpreted these changes to be the reason for the airline's decreasing profits. Webber hypothesized the fuel cost of flying Airbus A380 from Sydney to London in which he estimated the extra fuel cost at $472. Flying the airline in this route in both directions for a year meant incurring an additional fuel cost of $1 million. This additional cost accounts for 13% of Qantas profit. Following his investigations, Webber suggested that airlines should set a standard passenger weight to counter the increasing fuel cost. For instance, he gave an empirical weight of 75 kilograms as the standard weight. This implies that a passenger weighing 100 kilograms will be considered to be overweight by 25 kilograms, and this attracts a surcharge of $29 to fly from Sydney to London. On the other hand, a passenger with 50 kilograms body weight would be discounted the same amount. The second suggestion for Webber was to set a standard weight that will have passengers weighed on scales with their luggage, and then charged collectively (Singer, 2012).

This proposal gained immense popularity after Peter Singer, an ethicist supported Webber's idea by highlighting the reasons for introducing a 'pay-by-weight' system on airlines. Singer discussed the costs imposed to others by obese people, in order to justify as an ethical issue. In support of Webber's argument, Singer reaffirmed that people are getting fatter all over the world with developed countries carrying the highest burden of obesity. He sarcastically refers to the manner of movement associated to fat people as waddling rather than walking (Singer, 2012).

According to Singer, obesity has adverse consequences to the society, as well as the environment. Therefore, he agrees that surcharging passengers for extra weight will be a fair deal because it will reflect and individual's true cost of flight. In turn, the 'pay-by-weight' system will relieve fellow passengers from incurring extra costs on obese people. As such, Singer downplays the ethics that the new system is a discriminatory act. Ideally, Singer advocates for the introduction of public policies that discourage people from gaining weight, in order to reduce the extra cost imposed on others in the society. This is why he supports the 'pay-by-weight' system in the aviation industry.

Scientific inquiry has also exacerbated the debate on 'pay-by-weight' pricing policies on airlines. In November 2012, Bharat Bhatta, a Norway based economist published an article on the fat-taxes that aroused academic inquiry. Bhatta's approach was to solve the challenges involved in introducing the 'pay-by-weight' system in the aviation industry (Alemanno, 2013). In his article, he claimed that airlines do not exercise fairness in charging passengers under the current fare policy. This is so because all passengers pay an 'average price' regardless of their body weight. In this system, costs are distributed among passengers. This implies that passengers who have low weight such as 40 kilograms pay extra cost to compensate the extra weight of obese passengers. In order to address this indifference in cost distribution, Bhatta suggested that the adoption of the current fare policy on airlines will ensure that passengers pay based on their baggage. He suggested three principal approaches through which airlines can implement the new fare model. The first method is the adoption of price per kilogram charging that is considered as a straightforward approach. The second approach is surcharging heavier passengers and discounting the lighter ones, whereas the third method is setting fares in three bands of passengers as light, normal and heavy (Bhatta, 2013).

Case Scenario

Following these controversial perspectives, it seems some airlines are pleased by the idea of introducing the 'pay-by-weight' pricing policy. This aspect has been evidenced by the approach by Samoa Air. On April 1, 2013, Samoa Air announced what many people believed to be an April-pool joke. Contrary to the expectations of many, Samoa Air switched to the 'pay-by-weight' system. As such, it has become the first airline to adopt the new fare system in the world. Under the new fare system, the fare charged correlates with the passengers' weight and luggage, and this is considered as a fair deal (Davies, 2013).

According to critical analysis by aviation experts, this new system might work due to a number of reasons, but it appears unpractical for large airlines. One of the key reasons why 'pay-by-weight' system works with Samoa Air is that the airline operates short flight aircrafts. These aircrafts carry a dozen passengers; thus, logistical problems are not encountered in weighing each person. The second reason why the system might work with Samoa Air is the raising trends of obesity in the American Samoa region. It is reported that obesity has become an immense problem because two-thirds of the U.S. population is overweight or obese. Therefore, obesity has already become an ethical problem in the region. This implies that any public policy that seems to address the problems is reasonable. In this case, lightweight passengers are shielded from the adverse effects of obesity crisis in the region.

It is apparent that the adoption of the 'pay-by-weight' system by Samoa Air has created a tempting idea for other airlines. Some airlines are considering switching to the new fare system as one of the ways of recouping the extra fuel cost that seem to slim the profit margins. For instance, the 'customers of size' policy adopted by Southwest Airlines appears to be a replica of the 'pay-by-weight' policy. Under the 'customers of size' policy, the extra size of a passenger is determined by the armrests. Those who cannot fit between the armrests are considered to exceed the size of a conventional seat. As such, they are required to purchase another seat, in order to occupy a space of two seats (Davies, 2013).

Despite these approaches towards the adoption of the 'pay-by-weight' system, some airlines have expressed objection to it. For instance, EasyJet and Ryanair have already discarded the new idea (Davies, 2013). It is also likely that large carriers will not accept the new system because it is associated to an array of problems including legal and logistic issues.

Policies Related to 'Pay-by-Weight' Policy

Currently, there are no clearly communicated public policies related to obese passengers. In the United States, policies related to seats for obese people are set by airlines, but they are not protected by the constitutional law. This lack of a legal guideline on setting airline fares appears to be the most stabling block to the new approach of 'pay-by-weight' system. In contrast, rights of obese people are protected by most constitutions under the disability legislations. For instance, the Canadian judicial system prohibits discrimination based on body weight. In 2008, the Supreme Court ruled that imposing extra fares on passengers who are differently-abled is a form of discrimination. As such, obese people are considered to be among the differently-abled people. In its landmark ruling on extra fares, the court upheld the 'one person, one ticket' policy, implying that airlines do not have the right to surcharge obese passengers. This policy has become the mainstay of passenger services by airlines since the inception of commercial aviation (Funke, 2009).

The Right to be Fat

From a legal perspective, the Canadian case seems to be reflected in most countries. Despite the absence of body weight from the list of antidiscrimination provisions including Titles VII and XI of the Civil Rights Act and Equal Protection Clause, there are numerous implications of right to be fat. Under the precepts of current law, fatness has emerged in the legal discourse and culture as an identity that bears personality attributes. Tirosh (2013) reaffirms that "fatness emerges as a trait that allegedly reveals much more about the individual than medical information such as body mass index or fats in blood" (p. 280). This implies that, as sexuality, fatness falls under personality traits that are recognized by the law. This is probably the reason why most airlines and aviation experts view the 'pay-by-weight' pricing policy from the perspective of the underlying legal issues.

Legal Issue Case Related to 'Pay-by-Weight' Policy

It is apparent that overweight passengers might seek remedy in the Disability Act to challenge the 'pay-by-weight' policy expected to be imposed by airlines. An outstanding example of such cases can be provided by the Kenlie Tiggeman's case. In this case, the overweight passenger sued Southwest Airlines for discrimination. It is worth noting that Southwest Airline is one of the airlines that have adopted the new flight pricing system through what they refer to as the 'customers of size' policy. This case attracted immense public attention leading to the intervention of the district court that issued an injunction. In her application in the district court, Tiggeman claimed that the airline discriminates against obese customers. All these emerged from Southwest agents' response that she 'too fat to fly', requiring her to buy a second seat (Chang, Stuart, Effron & Sally, 2012).

Personal Reflection on the Ethical Dilemma

According to the turn of events, it is apparent that the issue of surcharging overweight passengers is surrounded by an ethical dilemma. Despite the facts associated with the proposal, it also raises immense controversy. For instance, it raises the question whether the 'pay-by-weight' approach will guarantee fairness than the status quo. On the other hand, the implementation of the new fare model seems to be hindered by both economical and technological issues. Moreover, it is still uncertain whether it would be logical to adopt the proposal. It is a popular assumption that the new pricing model that introduces price differentials serves as an incentive to passenger to lose weight, in order to pay reduced fares. If this would work, then it will play a significant role in addressing the obesity crisis. However, no such practice has existed in any transport mode. Therefore, this proposal is a new approach in the travel industry so its acceptance by the passengers and other stakeholders is compromised.

Conclusion

Conclusively, the issue of surcharging overweight passengers seems to be a good idea, especially when viewed from the economic perspective. According to the proposals by different experts, ranging from aviation economists to ethicists and environmental activists, flying overweight passenger has huge costs to the individual and society. Obesity is associated with health conditions that reduce the individual's quality of life. On the other hand, the society bears costs related to obesity population. In the case of airlines, flying obese people has been found to increase fuel cost. This translates to reduced profit margins for airlines. In the recent year, airlines have raised concern over the swelling obese population, especially in the developed countries including the United States, Australia, Canada, and the European Union states. As a result, some airlines have considered adopting a fare pricing model that will lift the burden of paying for extra cost incurred in flying obese people.

Historically, the idea of introducing 'pay-by-weight' policy, also called the 'fat-taxes' was conceived in the aviation industry through Tony Webber. His proposal was supported by Peter Singer who argued from the ethical side of the proposal. Later on, Bharat Bhatta published a controversial article that provided suggestions on how to implement the new pricing model. It is from these incidences that the debate emerged. Currently, some airlines have already adopted the 'pay-by-weight' policy, including Samoa Air and Southwest airlines. Ironically, Qantas, under which Webber worked as the senior economist has refused to adopt the new system.

From a legal perspective, most airlines are hesitant to adopt the proposed pricing model due to obvious reasons. First, the system appears to be discriminating obese people, and that attracts legal measures. On the other hand, the policy is not defined through constitutional provisions. So far, judicial systems uphold the 'one person, one ticket' policy. Therefore, extensive scientific inquiry is needed to decide whether the 'pay-by-weight' policy is fairer than 'average price' policy.

References

Alemanno, A. (2013). *Airline 'fat taxes': the dilemmas of the 'pay as you weigh' airline pricing policies*. Retrieved from http://www.albertoalemanno.eu/articles/airlinesfattax

Bhatta, B. (2013). Pay-as-you-weigh pricing of an air ticket: economics and major issues for discussions and investigations. *Journal of Revenue & Pricing Management, 12,* 103-119. doi:10.1057/rpm.2012.47

Chang, J., Stuart, E., Effron, L., & Sally, H. (2012 May 3). 'Too fat to fly' passenger sues southwest airlines for 'discriminatory actions.' *ABC News.* Retrieved from http://abcnews.go.com/Travel/fat-fly-passenger-sues-southwest-airlines-discriminatory-actions/story?id=16271932

Davies, A. (2013). *How long until all airlines charge more for fat people?* Retrieved from http://www.businessinsider.com/will-big-airlines-charge-fat-passengers-extra-2013-4

Funke, R. D. (2009). *Obese airline passengers.* Retrieved from https://philosophy.tamucc.edu/readings/ethics/cases/obese-airline-passengers?destination=node%2F1909

Singer, P. (2012). *Why airlines should start charging overweight customers by the pound.* Retrieved from http://www.businessinsider.com/overweight-passengers-are-eating-up-the-airline-industrys-profits-2012-3

Thomas, A. (2011). *Soft landing: airline industry strategy, service, and safety.* New York, NY: Apress.

Tirosh, Y. (2013).The right to be fat. *Yale Journal of Health Policy, Law, and Ethics, 12*(2), 266-308.

YOUR KNOWLEDGE HAS VALUE

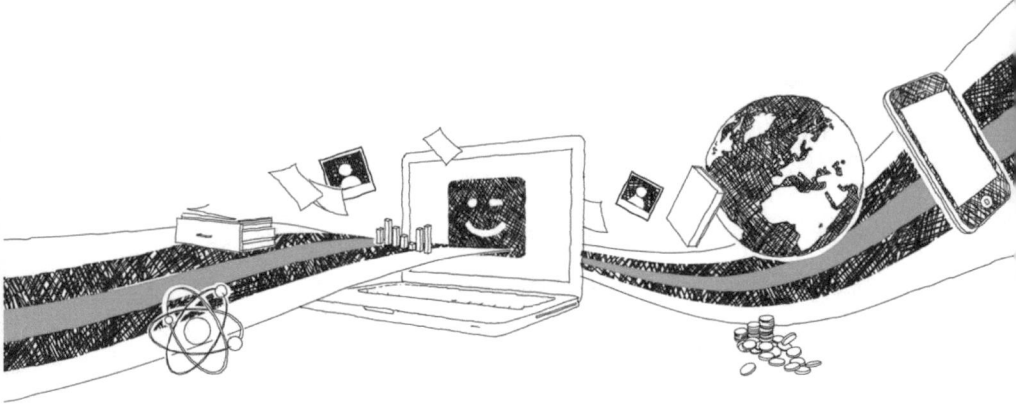

- We will publish your bachelor's and master's thesis, essays and papers

- Your own eBook and book - sold worldwide in all relevant shops

- Earn money with each sale

Upload your text at www.GRIN.com and publish for free

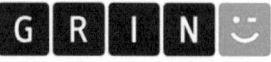